A Training Manual for the
Radiology Technologist
in the Vascular Access Center

Tonya L. McCree IVN R.T.

TLM Enterprise LLC
Akron

Copyright 2013 by TLM Enterprise, LLC
First Edition, 2013

Published in the United States of America

Warning—Disclaimer
This book is designed to provide information on your role as a Radiology Technologist. It is sold with the understanding that the publisher and author are not engaged in rendering medical advice. If medical and or other expert assistance is required, the services of a competent professional should be sought.
It is not the purpose of this manual to reprint all information that is otherwise available to authors and/ or publishers, but instead to complement, amplify and supplement other texts. You are urged to read all the available material, learn as much as possible about the Radiology Technologist in the Vascular Access Center and tailor the information to your individual needs. For more information, see the many resources in appendix 2.
Every effort has been made to make this manual as complete and as accurate as possible. However, there may be mistakes, both typographical and in content. Therefore, this text should be used only as a general guide and not as the ultimate source of information.
The purpose of this manual is to educate and assist. The author and TLM Enterprise shall have neither liability nor responsibility to any person or entity with respect to any loss or damage caused, or alleged to have been caused, directly or indirectly, by information contained in this book.

Matthew 7:7New International Version (NIV)

Ask, Seek, Knock
7 "Ask and it will be given to you; seek and you will find; knock and the door will be opened to you.

Contents

Foreword

This instructional manual will give you an understanding of your role as the Radiology Technologist in the **Vascular Access Center**. You will understand that each center is unique in size, procedures, supplies and job duties. This manual is designed with basic guidelines and helpful hints. In no way does this manual complete your training nor give a complete guide to all the responsibilities that may be expected of you. Additional training will come with on the job experience. As you read through this manual you will notice various words in bold print and their meaning can be found in the back of this manual under glossary. To personalize this manual for your specific needs use the provided space for further notes.

Chapter 1
Introduction to the Vascular Access Center

The Vascular Access Center is also known as the Interventional
Nephrology, Interventional Radiology and Dialysis Access Center.
Due to an increasing **Dialysis** patient population the Nephrologists
are treating their patients with interventional procedures. With the
use of Fluoroscopy and Ultrasound equipment the Interventional
Nephrologist can track and treat Dialysis patient in a timely
manner. The Vascular Access Center can accommodate the needs
of the dialysis patient with little to none interruptions in their
regular scheduled treatments. The program recognizes dialysis as
the first link to the patient's Lifeline.
By using sophisticated imaging equipment like **Fluoroscopy**,
interventional procedures in the Vascular Access Center are
possible. Specific techniques make many diseases treatable without
open surgical procedures. When using fluoroscopy equipment
extra rules do apply. Those rules are governed by the State in
which you preside. In Ohio for the example the regulations are
under the State of Ohio. The State of Ohio requires certification
for the facility and to the individuals performing service and
operating any radiation emitting equipment. By law Special
training and knowledge of emitting radiation doses to others is a
requirement. The State of Ohio requirements and regulations can
be found at www.odh.ohio.gov. The website is available to address
all radiation related questions. Specific safety measures are in
place to protect employees and individuals that will receive
radiation exposure. There are many sources available to assist
your individual questions and concerns.
 The Vascular Access Center has three very relevant positions: the
Interventional Nephrologist - a Physician specialized in
Nephrology who has completed a Fluoroscopy training program;
the Nurse with intravenous training with sedation experience and
the Radiology Technologist preferably with some interventional
background.

Each position has a very unique role in the Vascular Access Center. Each position relies on the other to perform his or her duties in order to be functional and successful. The procedures may be only diagnostic or they may include some interventional requirements. The staff, equipment and location will determine what procedures will be performed at the facility.

Procedure List
Fistulagram
Fistulagram with **Angioplasty**
Fistulagram with Angioplasty and **Stent**
Fistulagram with **Declot**
Vein Mapping
Temporary **Catheter** Placement
Temporary Catheter Removal
Permanent **Catheter** Placement
Permanent Catheter Exchange
Permanent Catheter Removal
Permanent Catheter Evaluation
Permanent Catheter Repair

Chapter 2
Value of the Radiology Technologist

The Radiology Technologist becomes one of the most valuable assets in the Vascular Access Center. The knowledge and skills of the Radiology Technologist will be used to assist and guide many processes. Management and organizational skills are key factors for success in the Interventional room. A Radiology Technologist that has experience in Special procedures or Cardiac Catheter Labs will be very helpful with expediting a smooth transition into the Vascular Access Center. Job duties for a Radiology Technologist are very similar from one lab to another which will expedite the training process. With a Special Procedures history you will maintain Radiology exposure factors, understand protocols for the sedated patient, and be well educated on equipment function and maintenance. You will know what type of supplies you need for every procedure and how to find vendors. You will understand the need for a consistent work flow and the importance of time. As an experienced Special Procedures Technologist you have some advantages in the Vascular Access Center. Radiology Technologist that does not have these skills is still qualified they will just need more time to adapt in the atmosphere.

Chapter 3
Qualification of the Radiology Technologist

Those Radiology Technologist interested in expanding their minds to more opportunities can make an easy transition into the Vascular Access Center. You will be the driving force that will wear many hats, but you will gain much knowledge. Your Radiology background will support the growing Interventional Nephrology foundation. You may be referred to as the Interventional Radiology Technologist, Dialysis Radiology Technologist, Vascular Access Radiology Technologist, the Chief Radiology Technologist and or the X-ray Technologist.

Objective   To obtain a position with career advancement opportunities that will enhance company goals.

Education   1988 University of Akron --- Akron, Ohio --- Associate Degree in Radiology Technology
    1985 Akron General Medical Center --- Akron, Ohio --- State Certified in Radiology Technology Member
    2009 Member of ASDIN American Society of Diagnostic & Interventional Nephrology
    2012 OSHA Compliance Workplace Safety
    2013 ACLS Advanced Cardiovascular Life Support Certification

Experience   October 2006 --- present: <u>Kidney & Hypertension Consultants</u> --- Canton, Ohio
    Chief Special Procedures Technologist, Education Outreach Coordinator
    Operate G.E. equipment, Scrub in with Nephrologists with sterile procedures, Radiation Safety Officer, Maintain Inventory, Sterilize Instruments, Manage Department Radiology Standards by maintaining all State Regulations, Certificate of completion NIH Office Research, Purchasing Manager using Peachtree Accounting System, Sales Representative Facilitator, Marketing and Education Coordinator, Physician Vascular Education Outreach Coordinator, Vascular Access Trainer
    June 2006 --- August 2006: <u>Parma Community Hospital</u> --- Parma, Ohio
    Special Procedures/ Diagnostic Technologist (First Assist Agency travel assignment)
    April 2005 --- February 2006: <u>Medina General Hospital</u> --- Medina, Ohio
    Diagnostic Radiology Technologist (First Assist Agency travel assignment)
    January 2005 --- February 2005: <u>Marymount Hospital</u> --- Cleveland, Ohio
    Cardiology Technologist (First Assist Agency travel assignment)
    November 2003 --- September 2004: <u>Cleveland Clinic Foundation</u> --- Cleveland, Ohio
    Vascular Interventional Radiology Technologist (First Assist Agency travel assignment)
    Prepare patients for interventional procedures, Obtain medical images
    using Siemens equipment responsible for new technician on -site training
    September 2003 --- November 2003: <u>Newton General Hospital</u> --- Atlanta, Georgia
    Cardiology/ Special procedures Technologist (Agency travel assignment)
    Assist in the Specials/ Cardiac Catheterization Lab on Phillips and G.E. Equipment
    Scrub and assist in Interventional procedures in Angiography and Cardiology

May 2003 --- August 2003: <u>St Vincent Charity Hospital</u> --- Cleveland,, Ohio

Diagnostic Radiology Technologist (First Assist Agency travel assignment)

Obtain radiographic images on inpatients and outpatients and emergency patients

Additional responsibilities include emergency room patients

January 2003 --- April; 2003: <u>Emory Healthcare</u> --- Atlanta, Georgia

Special Procedures Radiology Technologist (Maxim Agency travel assignment)

Prep patients for exams in the interventional department

Phillips equipment, PAX, Wet and Dry film processing

September 2002 --- December 2002: <u>Newton General Hospital</u> --- Covington, Georgia

Special Procedures/ Cardiac Catheterization Technologist (Agency travel assignment)

Perform interventional Angiography and Cardiology

Served as a Liaison between management and employees to facilitate communication

Responsible for developing operational procedures at the employee level

July 2002 --- September 2002: <u>Pittsburgh Children's Hospital</u> --- Pittsburgh, Pennsylvania

Special Procedures Radiology Technologist (Maxim Agency travel assignment)

Trained Co-workers on Toshiba Angiography unit/ Scrub procedures

November 1986 --- September 2002: <u>Summa Health Systems</u> --- Akron, Ohio

Special Procedures Technologist/ Diagnostic/ Mammography/ Diagnostic Supervisor/ Quality Control

Scheduling Technologist for Angiography, Operating room, Emergency and Diagnostic

Radiation Safety Coordinator, Experience on Siemens, Toshiba, G.E., Picker and Phillips equipment

Chapter 4
Interventional Nephrology Radiology Technologist

Why the Radiology Technologist?
As a certified Radiology Technologist you know the protocols for
x-ray exposure and understand the importance for **radiation
monitoring**.
You are familiar with the fast pace process because most x-rays are
time sensitive. Time sensitive procedures occur for patients
holding their breath for diagnostic x-rays to the speed of
angiography or **cine** film for **contrast** material. Radiology
Technologist learns about motion in the beginning phrases of
school. Radiology equipment and Radiology Technologist have a
connection and respect for knowing one cannot work without the
other. Just by the sound of the equipment you can usually tell if
there is a problem. You know the process for troubleshooting the
equipment and recognize when to call for service. The Radiology
Technologist stands as the center because the procedures are
dependent upon the fluoroscopy equipment. When the **C-arm**
works well, there are no interruptions in the flow of the schedule.
A Radiology Technologist must always be a step ahead.

Radiology Technologist

Perform a variety of complex specialized tasks eminent in operating radiographic equipment to perform Nephrology angiography, vascular interventional procedures in accordance with radiation safety procedures.
Set up sterile trays and other equipment practicing **sterile technique**.
Maintain a sterile environment
Safely position patients; immobilize as necessary
Operate Fluoroscopic equipment
Assist Nephrologists during angiography and interventional procedures to include handling of instruments, operating and monitoring equipment.
Scrub to assist with the passage of catheters, guide wires and other instruments needed for the procedure.
Process film, collate in sequence and label appropriately
Maintain film archival system
Schedule patient procedures
Document patients for procedures and supplies
Assist to improve education and training to other technologist
Maintain records and statistical data
Perform other related duties incidental to the work therein (patient transport, etc.)
Maintain supply inventory
Perform Purchasing Manager duties to order supplies
Perform Purchasing evaluations to maintain a cost effective budget
Perform Purchasing Consultant position with Sales Representatives
Negotiator for Equipment support contracts
Coordinate and be instrumental in collaborating training and conference classes
Physician Vascular Education Outreach Coordinator
Educate clients on Vascular Access Center
Marketing visits to create a relationship with potential clients
Assist Nephrologists with the development of new protocols and imaging techniques
Participate in research initiatives

Maintain Radiation Safety protocols

Educate employees / co-workers on Radiation protection

Radiation Safety Officer monitors all radiation badge readings and control devices

Annually review, train and monitor the compliance plan and privacy policy

Annually review all policies and procedures of the Dialysis Access Radiation Department

Annually train and certify all employees on Radiation safety and equipment

Annually review Ohio Department of Health policies and procedures

OSHA Safety Officer

Attend OSHA seminars

Annually review and update all OSHA policies and procedures

Train and certify all employees on OSHA compliance

Certification in National Institute of Health of Extramural Research

Maintain requirements **BLS** status

Maintain requirements for **ARRT** certification

Maintain requirements for Ohio Radiology License

<u>Specifics for Radiology Technologist only</u>

Perform a variety of complex specialized tasks eminent in operating radiographic equipment to perform Nephrology angiography, vascular interventional procedures in accordance with radiation safety procedures.

   a. Every morning you start off with a sign off sheet to acknowledge your radiation equipment is operational.

   b. Patient information must be entered into the C-arm equipment. Place patient label in radiation documentation book and complete when procedure is finish.

Set up sterile trays and other equipment practicing **sterile technique**. Maintain a sterile environment. When assisting the Doctor you will dress in sterile attire no outdoor clothing is permitted in procedure room. (Scrub uniform, bouffant or surgical cap, mask and shoe covers). You will use sterile protocol for setting up your tray and assisting the Doctor. Goggles may be used as an extra **PPE**. You can now proceed with a sterile scrub and then dress into the sterile gown and sterile gloves.

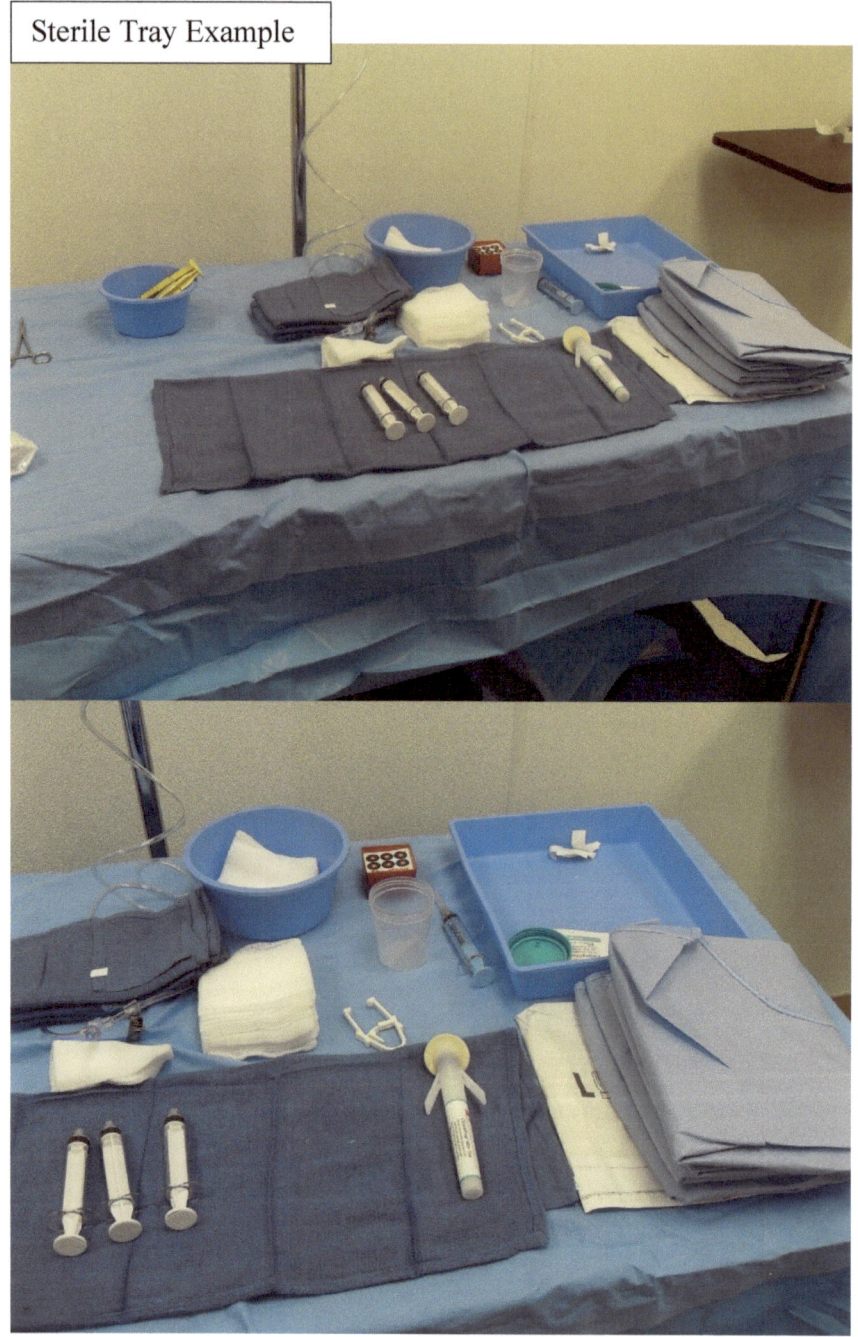

Sterile Tray Example

Prepping the patient

Catheter placement
Clean chest from sternum to arm pit.
Clean neck from ear lobe to nipple
Square off sterile area with blue towels
Fix sterile drape along pattern of towels cross over at the jaw area
Gather drapes and clamp to form a pocket around shoulder area

Fistulagram
Clean fistula site
Clean upper and lower arm from wrist to shoulder
Have patient raise arm and clean the underside.
Wrap the patients hand in sterile towel
Have patient raise arm and slide u drape under shoulder area
Starting with the foot side wrap drape around arm and then with the head side cross over drape toward the chest and finish wrapping the arm.
Gather drapes on top of the wrist area loosely and clamp this should allow the drapes to form a pocket on the radial and ulna side of the arm. (The pocket should risible a trough)
Always clamp sterile drape sheet to the u drape safely position patients; immobilize as necessary

Note to remember: Always flush anything with end holes.
Designate a specific place on the tray for all sharps.

Safely position patients and immobilize as necessary. Use safety devices like table straps to secure the patient. Most procedure tables have straps.

When operating the Fluoroscopic equipment remember low dose radiation factors for the entire room.

Assist Nephrologists during angiography and interventional procedures to include handling of instruments, operating and monitoring equipment. Scrub to assist with the passage of catheters, guide wires and other instruments needed for the procedure. Always remember once in the **scrub** position things must be arranged appropriately to maintain a sterile environment and still allow the Radiology Technologist to run the equipment.

Diagrams for positioning the room

White arrow C-arm fluoroscopy
Blue C-arm fluoroscopy monitor
Black X-ray exam table
Green Sterile tray table
Red Ultrasound machine
Orange Arm board

Right Catheter Placement

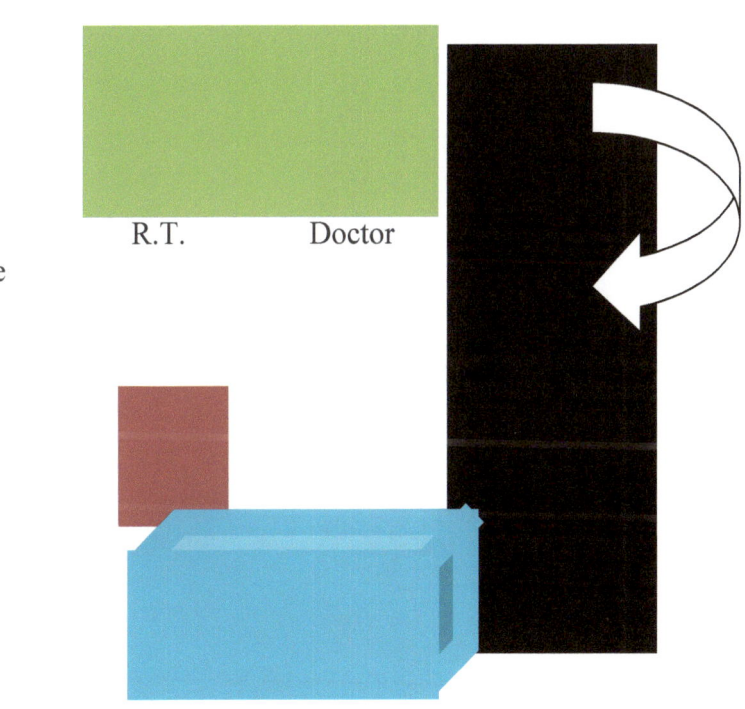

R.T.   Doctor

Nurse

Left catheter placement

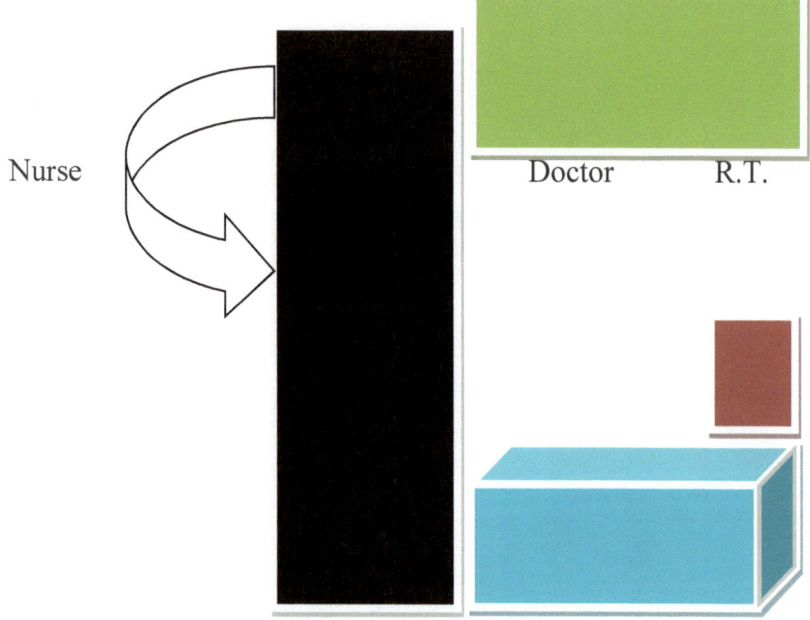

Nurse

Doctor   R.T.

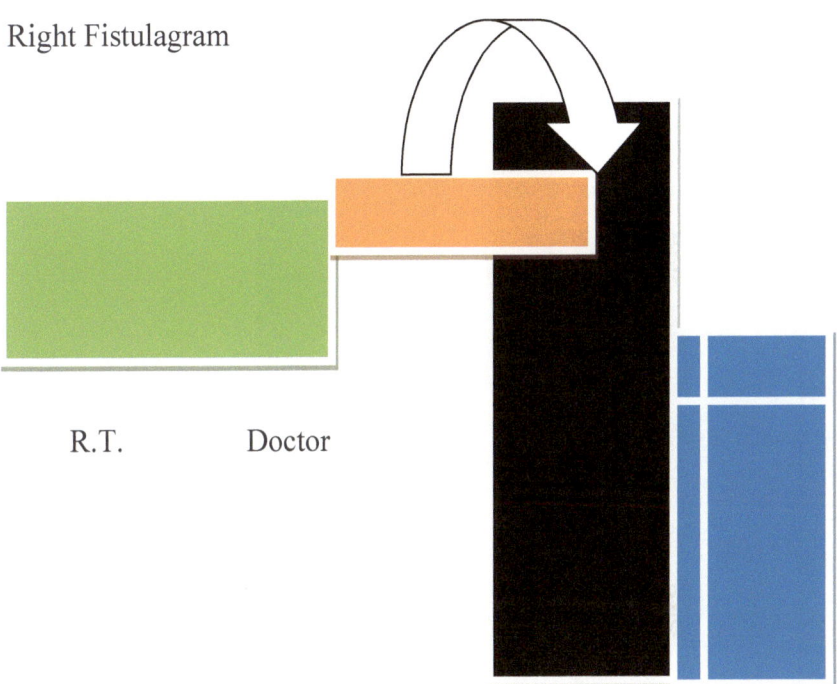
Right Fistulagram

R.T.   Doctor

Left Fistulagram

Nurse

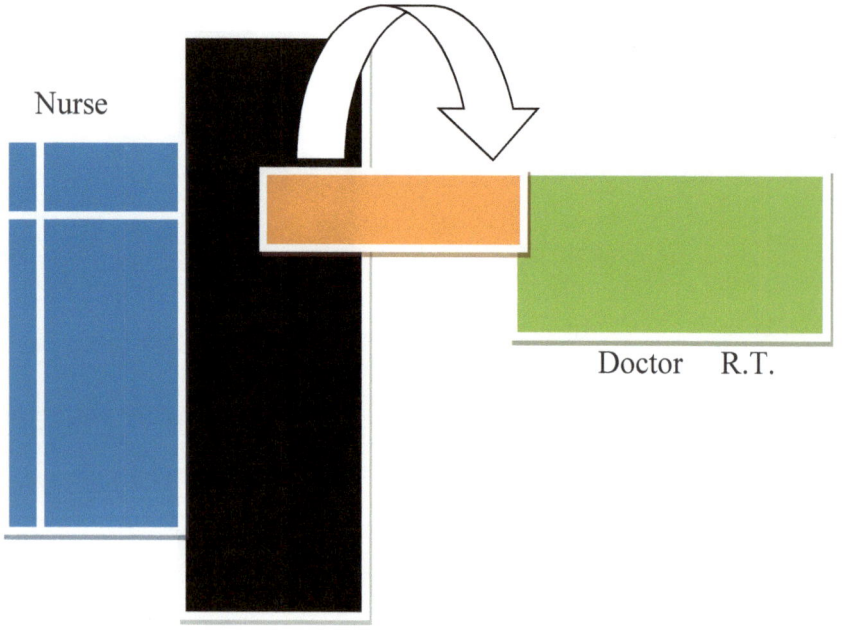

Doctor   R.T.

Process film/ burn disc, collate in sequence and label appropriately. Maintain film archival system. Record and document the request for release of medical imaging

Schedule patients for appropriate procedures and give pre and post procedure instructions.

Maintain a tracking system for supplies used for all procedures. Include serial numbers and dates for **implantable** supplies

Chapter 5
Extracurricular for the Radiology Technologist

Training is an essential element. You train others for the cohesiveness of the lab. The legal boundary of the Radiology room/equipment puts you in the chief position for how things flow in the procedure room. Your license requires you to be responsible for all that happens within those leaded walls.

Required Checks

Leaded Aprons checked annually
C-arm PM/Service log
Physicist logs
Radiation Monitor Program
Lead shielding checks
Safety of all personnel
Use of proper exposure techniques
Recording of all exposure
Weight limitations
Imaging process
Safe keeping of recorded images

Chapter 6
Beneficial Advice

Know the difference between major and minor supplies.

Tray packs help with time control. You may want to consider tray procedure packs. Packs are the quick set up without opening everything individually and you can custom to your needs.

Behind the scenes supplies are those things that are needed for everyday operation. Supplies that may not seem important are the very supplies that built the foundation of the company.

Foundation
Foundational things include the building of the lead walls to everything that is stored and placed in cabinets and on shelves. These items can be called miscellaneous but the make life easier.

Major and minor equipment should all have a check system in place. Establish a material management team to do minor repairs and annual check. Standardize a routine mail out processing for equipment quality checks.

Major equipment include

C-arm with subtraction and image storing
Radiation protective shields
Ultrasound is a standard for vein and fistula location and sizing
(with Doppler and color flow could be helpful)
X-ray table that can rise, lower and tilts head and foot. A table with
an arm rest and a safety strap (always be aware of table capacity)
Monitor for patient vital signs throughout procedure
Crash cart is required for EEG, EKG, and Emergency Medical
Defibrillator
Oxygen tank for those patients requiring O2
Autoclave to sterilize instruments for surgical procedures
Metal scrub table

(Extras may include a hopper if not using an enclosed system on
tray and a scrub sink for Doctor Prep)

Minor equipment include
Hand Held **Doppler** used to access the sound of the fistula
Glucose monitors to check blood sugar
(Extras may include a Blanket warmer for patient comfort. Rooms
could be set up with two sets of lights one being a dimmer switch.

ELECTRICAL EQUIPMENT CHECKS RESPONSIBILITY OF THE RADIOLOGY TECHNOLOGIST

FLUOROSCOPY C-ARM EQUIPMENT (SERVICE CONTRACT)
FLUOROSCOPY TABLE
ULTRASOUND MACHINE
EKG MONITOR WITH BLOOD PRESSURE AND PULSE OX
DEFIBRILLATOR WITH EMERGENCY CART
AUTOCLAVE INSTRUMENT STERILIZER
SCRUB SINK WITH RINSE BASIN FOR SURGICAL EQUIPMENT
SURGICAL LIGHT
REFRIGERATOR
SUCTION MACHINE
PROCEDURE ELECTRICAL OUTLETS

Chapter 7
Refining your Skills

Be prepared for the unexpected events. Always take in consideration the possibility of things not going as planned. Some Vascular Access Centers are not connected to a Hospital or near an Emergency facility.
Emergency stand-by items will allow time to for the EMS to arrive.
In conjunction to the emergency cart **Chest Tubes** and **Stents** will offer substantial support to the patient.

Always keep you your Emergency Activation process updated
Maintain and review State Regulations for your facility
Time and Safety are key points in the Vascular Access Center.

 Growing industries require staying updated on the new cutting edge procedures and equipment. Keep a good relationship with your sales representatives and stay up to date with the last supplies. There are many supplies that may come from many different vendors. You will scale down your inventory as you find the things that work best for you. Your routine will include things like skin cleansers, guide wires, access needles, sutures, catheters and many more items listed in helpful hints to set up your tray.

To get you started use the **helpful hints to set up your tray**

<u>Fistulagram</u>
Tray
Sterile Gloves
Extension tubing
Tegaderm (small)
Lidocaine 4cc
500cc NaChl
18 gage Access need
Guide wire
Contrast

<u>Fistulagram with angioplasty and</u>
<u>declot</u>
Tray
Sterile Gloves
Extension tubing
Tegaderm (small x 3)
18gage Needle
Guide wire
5 Fr Sheath
6 Fr Sheath
Lidocaine 6cc
500cc NaChl
Angioplasty balloon
Inflation device
4 Fr Fogarty
Scissors
Pick-ups
Needle driver
Non-absorbable suture
Contrast

<u>Vein mapping</u>
Non-Sterile gloves x 2
Gauze
Ext Tubing
Stopcock
20cc syringe (x 2)
10cc syringe (x 2)
Blue bowl x 2
Tape
Lead markers
250cc NaChl
Contrast

<u>Fistulagram with angioplasty</u>
Tray
Sterile Gloves
Extension tubing
Tegaderm (small x 2)/ Bandaids
18 gage needle
Guide wire
6 Fr Sheath
Lidocaine 4cc
500cc NaChl
Angioplasty balloon
Inflation device
Scissors
Pick-ups
Needle driver
Non-absorbable suture
Contrast

Catheter placement
Tray
Sterile Gloves
Micropuncture set
Ultrasound probe cover
Dialysis long-term Catheter kit
500cc NaChl
Large Tegaderm
Curved Hemostat
Scissors
Pick- ups
Needle driver
Non-absorbable suture
Absorbable suture
Steri Strips
Antibiotic ointment
Lidocaine 20cc

Temp Catheter placement
Tray
Sterile Gloves
Micropuncture set
Ultrasound probe cover
Dialysis temporary Catheter
500cc NaChl
Large Tegaderm
Scissors
Needle driver
Non-absorbable suture
Antibiotic ointment
Lidocaine 10cc

Catheter Evaluation
Tray
Sterile Gloves
500cc NaChl
Guide wire
Tegaderm

Catheter Exchange
Tray
Sterile Gloves
Guide wire
Micropuncture set
Catheter
500cc NaChl
Tegaderm
Curved Hemostat
Scissors
Pick- ups
Needle driver
Non-absorbable suture
Absorbable suture
Antibiotic ointment
Lidocaine 20cc

Catheter removal
*Tranpac (suture cabinet-ask Dr. 1st)
Table drape
Sterile gloves
Chloraprep
Lidocaine 4cc
10 cc syringe
18 ga. Needle
26 ga. Needle
4x4 Gauze
Suture removal kit
Curved hemostats x 2
Sterile towels x 3
Antibiotic ointment
Tegaderm

Catheter repair
Under pad
Sterile gloves
Sterile Towels x2
Catheter repair kit
Skin cleanser

Chapter 8
Resources

American Radiology Technology**www.arrt.org**
American Society Radiology Technology **www.asrt.org**
Bible Gateway www.biblegateway.com
Encyclopedia www.encyclopedia.com
Ohio Department Health Radiation Protection www.odh.ohi.gov

Chapter 9
Glossary

Angiography / Cine - medical imaging technique used to visualize
the inside, or lumen, of blood vessels and organs of the
body, with particular interest in the arteries, veins and the
heart chambers. This is traditionally done by injecting a
radiopaque contrast agent into the blood vessel and imaging
it by using x-ray based techniques such as fluoroscopy.
Vascular Access Center- is a facility with specific care
focused on the dialysis patient's needs.

Angioplasty - the repair of a blood vessel, as by inserting a
balloon-tipped catheter to unclog it or by replacing part of the
vessel with either a piece of the patient's own tissue or a prosthetic
device

ARRT - American Registry Radiology Technologist

Autoclave -an apparatus in which steam under pressure effects
sterilization.

BLS - basic life support

C-arm - the fluoroscopy equipment used in the surgical procedure
rooms

Catheter -tube shaped medical device used for exchanging blood to
and from the dialysis machine. The device may be temporary or
permanent.

Chest Tube - a flexible plastic tube that is inserted through the
chest wall and into the pleural space or mediastinum. It is used to
remove air (pneumothorax) or fluid (pleural effusion, blood), or
pus (empyema) from the intra-thoracic space.

Contrast - medium used to distinguish structures or fluids within a body.

Declot – procedure performed to remove a blood clot

Dialysis - is a process for removing waste and excess water from the blood, and is used primarily as an artificial replacement for lost kidney function in people with renal failure.

Doppler - an ultrasound device to listen to the flow of a vessel. May have different options like color flow

Fistulagram - an x-ray procedure to look at the blood flow and check for narrowed or blocked areas in a fistula/graft.

Fluoroscopy - is an imaging technique that uses X-rays to obtain real-time moving images of the internal structures of a patient through the use of a fluoroscope. The images are then recorded and played on a monitor.

Implantable – a material, foreign to the body, surgical insertion under the skin for access or control.

Interventional Nephrologist - a physician who is an expert in nephrology who has taken additional training to maintain and improve vascular access for hemodialysis patients with the assistance of the fluoroscopy equipment. They study normal kidney function, kidney problems, the treatment of kidney problems and renal replacement therapy.

OSHA - occupational safety and health administration

PPE - personal protective equipment used to reduce employee exposure to hazards.

Radiation Monitoring - is tracking the calculation and assessment of the ionizing radiation dose received by the human body due to both external irradiation and the ingestion or inhalation of radioactive materials. Tracking is extensively for radiation protection and is routinely applied to occupational radiation workers, where a radiation dose is expected.

Radiation Safety Officer - individual the oversee the radiation monitoring

Scrub - knowledge and skills in sterile and aseptic techniques

Stent - medication device used to maintain the opening of a vessel

Sterile technique - a matter used in which to maintain an environment free of contaminants.

Ultrasound - The use of ultrasonic waves for diagnostic or therapeutic purposes, specifically to visualize an internal body structure.

Vascular Access Center - Interventional Physicians and specialized staff dedicated to the care and treatment of patients with Kidney Disease.

Vein mapping - the injection of contrast material into the venous system to determine the most sufficient veins, to form a fistula for dialysis treatments

A Training Manuel for the Radiology Technologist
working in the
Vascular Access Center

This Manual will serve as a resource to enhance your existing knowledge and skills as a Radiology Technologist.

Outstanding Features:
Easy to read
Well illustrated diagrams
Outlined with extra space for additional notes

The Vascular Access Center is helping the Nephrology Physicians,
     to
expedite treatment plans which allow for better outcomes. With
     the
growing population of Dialysis cases, this manual is a great
     reference.
Radiology Technologist can use this manual, to assist
the Nephrologists with interventional procedures.

About the Author

Tonya L. McCree R.T. is a Chief Radiology Technologist for a Vascular Access Center. For over 25 years of experience, she has gained knowledge and specialty skills in Diagnostic Radiology, Mammography, Angiography, Cardiology and Interventional Nephrology. Working in a Vascular Access Center has allowed her the
opportunity of the Scrub Tech., Radiation Safety Officer, Education
Outreach Coordinator and Purchasing Manager.